49 Headache and Migraine Juicing Solutions:

Stop Migraines and Headaches in a Matter of Days without Pills or Medical Treatments

By

Joe Correa CSN

COPYRIGHT

© 2017 Live Stronger Faster Inc.

All rights reserved

Reproduction or translation of any part of this work beyond that permitted by section 107 or 108 of the 1976 United States Copyright Act without the permission of the copyright owner is unlawful.

This publication is designed to provide accurate and authoritative information in regard to the subject matter covered. It is sold with the understanding that neither the author nor the publisher is engaged in rendering medical advice. If medical advice or assistance is needed, consult with a doctor. This book is considered a guide and should not be used in any way detrimental to your health. Consult with a physician before starting this nutritional plan to make sure it's right for you.

ACKNOWLEDGEMENTS

This book is dedicated to my friends and family that have had mild or serious illnesses so that you may find a solution and make the necessary changes in your life.

49 Headache and Migraine Juicing Solutions:

Stop Migraines and Headaches in a Matter of Days without Pills or Medical Treatments

By

Joe Correa CSN

CONTENTS

Copyright

Acknowledgements

About The Author

Introduction

49 Headache and Migraine Juicing Solutions: Stop Migraines and Headaches in a Matter of Days without Pills or Medical Treatments

Additional Titles from This Author

ABOUT THE AUTHOR

After years of Research, I honestly believe in the positive effects that proper nutrition can have over the body and mind. My knowledge and experience has helped me live healthier throughout the years and which I have shared with family and friends. The more you know about eating and drinking healthier, the sooner you will want to change your life and eating habits.

Nutrition is a key part in the process of being healthy and living longer so get started today. The first step is the most important and the most significant.

INTRODUCTION

49 Headache and Migraine Juicing Solutions: Stop Migraines and Headaches in a Matter of Days without Pills or Medical Treatments

By Joe Correa CSN

Headaches are a common problem people experience all the time during their life. Usually, they appear and disappear spontaneously not causing any serious problems or damage. In these cases, headaches are related to stress, problems with blood vessels, nervous system, physical inactivity, or problems with the muscles of the neck or eyes.

Knowing the difference between a headache and a migraine is extremely important because it can mean a better treatment method and prevent future pain from occurring in the first place.

Unlike traditional, low-intensity headaches that come and go without any pattern, migraines are more painful and is often a more severe type of headache. It's followed by some standard symptoms that include nausea, vomiting, sensitivity to light behind one eye or ear, and even temporary vision loss. In some cases, people experience such severe headaches that they are hospitalized.

Some people tend to develop migraine patterns that appear a couple of days before a headache occurs. This phenomenon is known as the 'prodrome' phase and includes irritability, different food cravings, yawning, depression, neck stiffness, and constipation. Combined with severe migraine headaches, these symptoms affect quality of life and should be treated.

Seeking professional medical care is a priority when dealing with headaches and/or migraines. Your physician will determine the definite cause of your problems and prescribe the correct treatment. There are, however, certain things you can do for yourself to prevent the pain. Some foods like fresh fruits and vegetables, leafy greens, rice and whole grains have proven to prevent or at least ease a headache and migraine.

As someone who has been able to eliminate cronic headaches, I have found that eating plenty of fresh fruits and vegetables every single day helped me put things under control. Also, increase water consumption and reduce red meat consumption.

The easiest way to get the right amount of foods is definitely a fresh homemade juice without any unhealthy additives or sugars.

That's how I came up with the idea to create this collection of migraine and headache preventing juice recipes. It's the easiest, the fastest, and the least expensive way to give your body a daily dose of precious vitamins and minerals, clean your body, and prevent sudden headaches.

Preparing these juices every day will mean a happier and healthier life, without constant headaches, migraines, or any other symptoms related to these conditions. Get started and see the results sooner than you can imagine!

49 HEADACHE AND MIGRAINE JUICING SOLUTIONS: STOP MIGRAINES AND HEADACHES IN A MATTER OF DAYS WITHOUT PILLS OR MEDICAL TREATMENTS

1. Cabbage Apple Juice

Ingredients:

1 cup of green cabbage, torn

1 small Granny Smith's apple, cored

2 cups of broccoli, chopped

1 cup of cauliflower, chopped

¼ tsp of turmeric, ground

2 oz of water

Preparation:

Wash the cabbage thoroughly under cold running water and drain. Torn into small pieces and set aside.

Wash the apple and cut lengthwise in half. Remove the core and cut into bite-sized pieces. Set aside.

Wash the broccoli and trim off the outer layers. Chop into small pieces and fill the measuring cup. Reserve the rest for later.

Wash the cauliflower and trim off the outer leaves. Chop into small pieces and fill the measuring cup. Reserve the rest in the refrigerator.

Rinse the onion stalk and chop into small pieces. Set aside.

Now, combine cabbage, apple, broccoli, and cauliflower in a juicer and process until juiced.

Transfer to a serving glass and stir in the turmeric and water. Refrigerate for 5 minutes before serving.

Nutrition information per serving: Kcal: 142, Protein: 8.9, Carbs: 42.2g, Fats: 1.3g

2. Apple Kiwi Juice

Ingredients:

1 Red Delicious apple, cored and chopped

1 whole kiwi, peeled and chopped

1 cup of blueberries

1 whole lemon, halved

¼ tsp of ginger, ground

1 oz of water

Preparation:

Wash the apple and cut lengthwise in half. Remove the core and cut into bite-sized pieces and set aside.

Peel the kiwi and cut into small pieces. Make sure to reserve the kiwi juice while cutting.

Place the blueberries in a colander. Rinse well under cold running water and drain. Fill the measuring cup and reserve the rest in the refrigerator.

Peel the lemon and cut lengthwise in half. Set aside.

Now, combine apple, kiwi, blueberries, and lemon in a juicer and process until juiced. Transfer to a serving glass and stir in the ginger, water, and reserved kiwi juice.

Add some crushed ice and serve immediately.

Nutrition information per serving: Kcal: 217, Protein: 3.2g, Carbs: 66.2g, Fats: 1.3g

3. Green Coconut Juice

Ingredients:

1 cup of beet greens, torn

1 cup of kale, chopped

1 cup of parsley, chopped

2 small cucumbers, peeled

1 whole lime, peeled and halved

1 tbsp of agave syrup

3 tbsp of coconut water

Preparation:

Combine beet greens, kale, and parsley in a large colander. Rinse under cold running water and drain. Chop into small pieces and set aside.

Wash the cucumber and cut into thin slices. Set aside.

Peel the lime and cut lengthwise in half. Set aside.

Now, combine beet greens, kale, parsley, cucumber, and lime in a juicer. Process until juiced. Transfer to a serving glass and stir in the agave and coconut water.

Mix well and serve cold.

Nutrition information per serving: Kcal: 139, Protein: 10.6g, Carbs: 42.2g, Fats: 1.9g

4. Pear Raspberry Juice

Ingredients:

3 large pears, cored and chopped

1 cup of fresh raspberries

1 medium-sized beet, trimmed

1 large lemon, peeled

1 oz of water

Preparation:

Wash the pear and cut in half. Remove the core and cut into bite-sized pieces. Set aside.

Rinse the raspberries in a colander and drain. Set aside.

Wash the beet and trim off the green parts. Peel and chop into bite-sized pieces. Set aside.

Peel the lemon and cut lengthwise in half. Set aside.

Now, combine pear, raspberries, beet, and lemon in a juicer. Process until juiced.

Transfer to a serving glass and stir in the water. Add some crushed ice and serve immediately.

Nutrition information per serving: Kcal: 378, Protein: 2.7g, Carbs: 133g, Fats: 2.7g

5. Swiss Chard Apple Juice

Ingredients:

1 cup of Swiss chard, chopped

1 large green apple, cored

1 cup of fresh basil, chopped

1 large lemon, peeled

1 cup of fresh mint, chopped

2 oz of water

Preparation:

Combine basil, Swiss chard, and mint in a large colander. Wash thoroughly under cold running water. Chop into small pieces and set aside.

Wash the apple and cut in half. Remove the core and cut into bite-sized pieces. Set aside.

Peel the lemon and cut lengthwise in half.

Now, combine Swiss chard, apple, basil, mint, and lemon in a juicer and process until well juiced. Transfer to serving glasses and stir in the water.

Refrigerate for 5 minutes before serving.

Enjoy!

Nutrition information per serving: Kcal: 126, Protein: 3.9g, Carbs: 39.1g, Fats: 1.1g

6.   Carrot Watercress Juice

Ingredients:

2 large carrots, sliced

1 cup of watercress, torn

1 cup of pineapple, chunked

1 large lime, peeled

1 small ginger knob, peeled

2 oz of water

Preparation:

Wash and peel the carrots. Cut into thin slices and set aside.

Wash the watercress thoroughly under cold running water. Torn with hands and set aside.

Cut the top of a pineapple and peel it with sharp cutting knife. Chop into small chunks and set aside.

Peel the lime and cut lengthwise in half. Set aside.

Peel the ginger root knob and cut into small pieces. Set aside.

Now, combine carrots, watercress, pineapple, lemon, and ginger in a juicer and process until well juiced.

Transfer to serving glasses and stir in water.

Add some ice and serve.

Nutrition information per serving: Kcal: 135, Protein: 3.3g, Carbs: 40.6g, Fats: 3.3g

7. Celery Turmeric Juice

Ingredients:

1 cup of celery, chopped

¼ tsp of turmeric, ground

1 cup of asparagus, trimmed

1 large green bell pepper, chopped

¼ tsp of ginger, ground

1 oz of water

Preparation:

Wash the celery and chop into small pieces. Set aside.

Wash the asparagus and trim off the woody ends. Cut into small pieces and fill the measuring cup. Reserve the rest in the refrigerator.

Wash the bell pepper and cut lengthwise in half. Remove the stem and seeds. Chop into small pieces and set aside.

Now, combine celery, asparagus, pepper, in a juicer and process until well juiced. Transfer to a serving glass and stir in the turmeric, ginger, and water.

Add some ice and serve immediately.

Enjoy!

Nutrition information per serving: Kcal: 48, Protein: 5.1g, Carbs: 15.8g, Fats: 0.6g

8. Apple Asparagus Juice

Ingredients:

1 large Granny Smith's apple, cored

1 cup of fresh asparagus, trimmed

3 medium-sized oranges, peeled and wedged

¼ tsp of turmeric, ground

2 oz of water

Preparation:

Peel the oranges and divide into wedges. Set aside.

Wash the apple and remove the core. Cut into bite-sized pieces and set aside.

Wash the asparagus thoroughly under cold running water and trim off the woody ends. Cut into small pieces and set aside.

Now, combine apple, asparagus, and oranges in a juicer and process until juiced. Transfer to serving glasses and stir in the turmeric and water.

Refrigerate for 5 minutes before serving.

Nutrition information per serving: Kcal: 316, Protein:

9.1g, Carbs: 98.1g, Fats: 1.2g

9. Pear Pepper Juice

Ingredients:

1 large pear, cored and chopped

1 large red bell pepper, chopped

2 cups of beets, chopped

1 large lemon, peeled

1 small ginger root slice, peeled

2 oz of water

Preparation:

Wash the pear and cut in half. Remove the core and cut into bite-sized pieces. Set aside.

Wash the bell pepper and cut in half. Remove the seeds and cut into small pieces. Set aside.

Wash the beets and trim off the green ends. Cut into small pieces and fill the measuring cup. Reserve the greens for some other juice. Set aside.

Peel the lemon and cut lengthwise in half. Set aside.

Peel the ginger slice and cut in half. Set aside.

Now, combine pear, bell pepper, beets, lemon, and ginger in a juicer. Process until well juiced and transfer to serving glasses.

Stir in the water and add some ice before serving.

Enjoy!

Nutrition information per serving: Kcal: 239, Protein: 7.5g, Carbs: 76.7g, Fats: 1.4g

10. Avocado Kale Juice

Ingredients:

1 cup of avocado, cubed

1 cup of fresh kale, torn

2 cups of Iceberg lettuce, torn

1 whole kiwi, peeled and halved

1 whole cucumber, sliced

Preparation:

Peel the avocado and cut lengthwise in half. Remove the pit and cut into small cubes. Fill the measuring cup and reserve the rest for later.

Combine kale and lettuce in a large colander. Wash thoroughly under cold running water and torn into small pieces. Set aside.

Peel the kiwi and cut lengthwise in half. Set aside.

Wash the cucumber and cut into thin slices. Fill the measuring cup and reserve the rest for later.

Now, combine avocado, kale, lettuce, kiwi, and cucumber in a juicer and process until juiced. Transfer to a serving glass and add some ice before serving.

Enjoy!

Nutrition information per serving: Kcal: 304, Protein: 9.8g, Carbs: 42.8g, Fats: 23.6g

11. Spinach Watercress Juice

Ingredients:

2 cups of spinach, torn

1 cup of watercress, torn

1 cup of kale, torn

1 cup of Swiss chard, torn

¼ tsp of ginger, ground

1 oz of water

Preparation:

Combine, spinach, watercress, kale, and Swiss chard in a large colander. Wash thoroughly under cold running water. Slightly drain and torn into small pieces.

Now, transfer the greens to a juicer and process until juiced. Transfer to a serving glass and stir in the ginger and water.

Refrigerate for 10 minutes before serving.

Enjoy!

Nutrition information per serving: Kcal: 87, Protein: 16.3g, Carbs: 22.9g, Fats: 2.4g

12. Banana Apple Juice

Ingredients:

1 cup of pomegranate seeds

1 large banana, chopped

1 small Granny Smith's apple, cored

1 cup of raspberries

¼ tsp of ginger, ground

Preparation:

Peel the banana and cut into small pieces. Set aside.

Wash the apple and cut lengthwise in half. Remove the core and cut into bite-sized pieces. Set aside.

Cut the top of the pomegranate fruit using a sharp paring knife. Slice down to each of the white membranes inside of the fruit. Pop the seeds into a measuring cup and set aside.

Rinse the raspberries under cold running water using a colander. Drain and set aside.

Now, combine banana, apple, pomegranate seeds, and raspberries in a juicer and process until juiced. Transfer to a serving glass and stir in the ginger.

Add some ice and serve immediately.

Nutrition information per serving: Kcal: 265, Protein: 5.1g, Carbs: 81.6g, Fats: 2.5g

13. Blackberry Mint Juice

Ingredients:

1 cup of blackberries

1 cup of fresh mint, chopped

1 whole lime, peeled

1 cup of pineapple, chunked

2 oz of coconut water

Preparation:

Place the blackberries in a large colander. Rinse thoroughly under cold running water. Drain and set aside.

Wash the mint and drain. Chop into small pieces and set aside.

Peel the lime and cut lengthwise in half. Set aside.

Using a sharp paring knife, cut the top of the pineapple. Gently remove all hard skin and slice it into thin slices. Fill the measuring cup and reserve the rest for later.

Now, combine blackberries, mint, lime, and pineapple in a juicer. Process until well juiced and transfer to a serving glass.

Stir in the coconut water and add few ice cubes before serving. Enjoy!

Nutrition information per serving: Kcal: 125, Protein: 4g, Carbs: 42.9g, Fats: 1.2g

14.   Orange Grape Juice

Ingredients:

1 large red orange, peeled

1 cup of green grapes

1 cup of beets, trimmed and sliced

1 whole apricot, pitted

1 tbsp of coconut water

Preparation:

Peel the orange and divide into wedges. Cut each wedge in half and set aside.

Rinse the grapes and remove the stems. Set aside.

Wash the beets and trim off the green parts. Cut into thin slices and fill the measuring cup. Reserve the rest for later.

Wash the apricot and cut lengthwise in half. Remove the pit and cut into small pieces. Set aside.

Now, combine orange, grapes, beets, and apricots in a juicer and process until well juiced. Transfer to a serving glass and stir in the coconut water.

Add some ice and serve immediately.

Nutrition information per serving: Kcal: 184, Protein: 4.9g, Carbs: 54.3g, Fats: 0.9g

15. Lemon Watermelon Juice

Ingredients:

1 whole lemon, peeled

1 cup of watermelon, chunked

1 large pear, chopped

1 cup of cranberries

¼ tsp of cinnamon, ground

1 oz of water

Preparation:

Peel the lemon and cut lengthwise in half. Set aside.

Cut the watermelon in half. Cut one large wedge and wrap the rest in a plastic foil and refrigerate. Peel the slice and cut into small cubes. Remove the pits and fill the measuring cup. Set aside.

Wash the pear and cut in half. Remove the core and cut into small pieces. Set aside.

Place the cranberries in a colander and rinse under cold running water. Drain and set aside.

Now, combine lemon, watermelon, pear, and cranberries

in a juicer and process until well juiced. Transfer to a serving glass and stir in the cinnamon and water.

Refrigerate for 5 minutes before serving.

Nutrition information per serving: Kcal: 186, Protein: 2.8g, Carbs: 64.1g, Fats: 0.8g

16. Plum Cantaloupe Juice

Ingredients:

1 whole plum, chopped

1 cup of cantaloupe, chopped

1 large orange, peeled

1 cup of fresh mint, torn

¼ tsp of ginger, ground

Preparation:

Wash the plum and cut in half. Remove the pit and chop into small pieces. Set aside.

Cut the cantaloupe in half. Scoop out the seeds and flesh. Cut and peel one large wedge. Chop into chunks and fill the measuring cup. Reserve the rest of the cantaloupe in a refrigerator.

Peel the orange and divide into wedges. Cut each wedge in half and set aside.

Wash the mint thoroughly under cold running water. Torn into small pieces and set aside.

Now, combine orange, plum, cantaloupe, and mint in a

juicer and process until juiced. Transfer to a serving glass and stir in the ginger.

Add some ice and serve immediately.

Enjoy!

Nutrition information per serving: Kcal: 151, Protein: 4.4g, Carbs: 45.6g, Fats: 0.9g

17. Banana Lime Juice

Ingredients:

1 large banana, chopped

1 whole lime, peeled

1 cup of watermelon, chopped

1 cup of fresh mint, torn

1 small Granny Smith's apple, cored

¼ tsp of cinnamon, ground

Preparation:

Peel the banana and cut into small chunks. Set aside.

Peel the lime and cut lengthwise in half. Set aside.

Cut the watermelon in half. Cut one large wedge and wrap the rest in a plastic foil and refrigerate. Peel the slice and cut into small cubes. Remove the pits and fill the measuring cup. Set aside.

Wash the mint thoroughly under cold running water. Drain and torn into small pieces. Set aside.

Wash the apple and cut lengthwise in half. Remove the core and chop into bite-sized pieces. Set aside.

Now, combine banana, lime, watermelon, mint, and apple in a juicer and process until juiced. Transfer to a serving glass and stir in the cinnamon.

Add some crushed ice and serve immediately.

Nutrition information per serving: Kcal: 239, Protein: 4.2g, Carbs: 69.5g, Fats: 1.2g

18. Blackberry Apple Juice

Ingredients:

1 cup of blackberries

1 small Golden Delicious apple, cored

1 cup of strawberries, chopped

1 large pear, chopped

¼ tsp of cinnamon, ground

1 oz of water

Preparation:

Wash the blackberries using a colander. Drain and set aside.

Wash the apple and cut lengthwise in half. Remove the core and chop into bite-sized pieces. Set aside.

Wash the strawberries and remove the stems. Cut into small pieces and fill the measuring cup. Reserve the rest in the refrigerator.

Wash the pear and cut in half. Remove the core and cut into small pieces. Set aside.

Now, combine blackberries, apple, strawberries, and pear

in a juicer and process until well juiced. Transfer to a serving glass and stir in the cinnamon.

Refrigerate for 5 minutes before serving.

Enjoy!

Nutrition information per serving: Kcal: 246, Protein: 4.2g, Carbs: 82.1g, Fats: 1.7g

19. Fennel Apple Juice

Ingredients:

1 cup of fennel, chopped

1 small Granny Smith's apple, cored

1 large orange, peeled

1 cup of blueberries

¼ tsp of ginger, ground

Preparation:

Trim off the outer wilted layers of the fennel. Roughly chop it and fill the measuring cup. Reserve the rest for later.

Wash the apple and cut lengthwise in half. Remove the core and cut into bite-sized pieces. Set aside.

Peel the orange and divide into wedges. Cut each wedge in half and set aside.

Place the blueberries in a colander and wash thoroughly under cold running water. Drain and set aside.

Now, combine fennel, apple, orange, and blueberries in a juicer and process until juiced. Transfer to a serving glass and stir in the ginger.

Add few ice cubes and serve immediately.

Enjoy!

Nutrition information per serving: Kcal: 222, Protein: 4.5g, Carbs: 69.1g, Fats: 1.5g

20. Spinach Pomegranate Juice

Ingredients:

1 cup of fresh spinach, torn

1 cup of pomegranate seeds

1 cup of sweet potato, cubed

1 whole lemon, peeled

2 oz of water

Preparation:

Wash the spinach thoroughly under cold running water. Drain and torn into small pieces. Set aside.

Cut the top of the pomegranate fruit using a sharp paring knife. Slice down to each of the white membranes inside of the fruit. Pop the seeds into a measuring cup and set aside.

Peel the sweet potato and cut into small cubes. Place in a deep pot and add 3 cups of water. Bring it to a boil and cook for 5 minutes. Remove from the heat and drain. Set aside.

Peel the lemon and cut lengthwise in half. Set aside.

Now, combine spinach, pomegranate seeds, previously cooked potato, and lemon in a juicer. Process until well juiced.

Transfer to a serving glass and stir in the water. Add some ice and serve immediately.

Enjoy!

Nutrition information per serving: Kcal: 195, Protein: 10.2g, Carbs: 56.1g, Fats: 2.1g

21. Watermelon Banana Juice

Ingredients:

1 large wedge of watermelon

1 large banana, sliced

1 cup of strawberries, chopped

2 whole plums, pitted

Preparation:

Cut the watermelon in half. Cut one large wedge and wrap the rest in a plastic foil and refrigerate. Peel the slice and cut into small cubes. Remove the pits and fill the measuring cup. Set aside.

Peel the banana and cut into thin slices. Set aside.

Wash the strawberries and remove the stems. Cut into small pieces and fill the measuring cup. Reserve the rest for in the refrigerator.

Wash the plums and cut into halves. Remove the pits and cut into small pieces. Set aside.

Now, combine watermelon, banana, strawberries, and plums in a juicer and process until juiced. Transfer to a serving glass and add some ice.

Serve immediately.

Nutrition information per serving: Kcal: 273, Protein: 5.1g, Carbs: 78.8g, Fats: 1.6g

22.   Asparagus Collard Green Juice

Ingredients:

1 cup of asparagus, trimmed and chopped

1 cup of collard greens, torn

1 medium-sized tomato, chopped

1 cup of spinach, torn

¼ tsp salt

1 rosemary sprig

Preparation:

Wash the asparagus and trim off the woody ends. Cut into small pieces and fill the measuring cup. Set aside.

Combine collard greens and spinach in a large colander. Wash under cold running water and drain. Torn into small pieces and set aside.

Wash the tomato and place it in a small bowl. Cut into small pieces and reserve the tomato juice while cutting. Set aside.

Now, combine asparagus, collard greens, tomato, and spinach in a juicer and process until juiced. Transfer to a serving glass and stir in the reserve tomato juice and salt. Sprinkle with rosemary.

Serve immediately.

Nutrition information per serving: Kcal: 66, Protein: 11.2g, Carbs: 19.6g, Fats: 1.5g

23. Strawberry Apple Juice

Ingredients:

1 cup of strawberries, chopped

1 small Granny Smith's apple, cored and chopped

1 whole guava, chunked

1 whole lemon, peeled and halved

¼ tsp of cinnamon, ground

2 oz of water

Preparation:

Wash the strawberries and remove the stems. Cut into small pieces and fill the measuring cup. Reserve the rest in the refrigerator. Set aside.

Wash the apple and cut lengthwise in half. Remove the core and cut into bite-sized pieces. Set aside.

Peel the guava and cut in half. Scoop out the seeds and wash it. Cut into small chunks and set aside.

Peel the lemon and cut lengthwise in half. Set aside.

Now, combine strawberries, apple, guava, and lemon in a juicer and process until juiced. Transfer to a serving glass and stir in the cinnamon and water.

Refrigerate for 10 minutes before serving.

Enjoy!

Nutrition information per serving: Kcal: 136, Protein: 3.6g, Carbs: 43.9g, Fats: 1.3g

24. Lettuce Cabbage Juice

Ingredients:

1 cup of red leaf lettuce, chopped

1 cup of purple cabbage, chopped

1 medium-sized artichoke, chopped

1 cup of fresh basil, torn

1 cup of cucumber, sliced

1 large carrot, sliced

Preparation:

Combine lettuce and cabbage in a large colander and rinse well under cold running water. Drain and chop into small pieces. Set aside.

Trim off the outer layers of the artichoke using a sharp paring knife. Cut into bite-sized pieces and set aside.

Rinse the basil with cold water and torn into small pieces. Set aside.

Wash the cucumber and cut into thin slices. Fill the measuring cup and reserve the rest in the refrigerator.

Wash and peel the carrot. Cut into thin slices and set

aside.

Now, combine lettuce, cabbage, artichoke, basil, cucumber, and carrot in a juicer and process until juiced.

Transfer to a serving glass and serve immediately.

Nutrition information per serving: Kcal: 88, Protein: 7.6g, Carbs: 30.1g, Fats: 0.7g

25. Cherry Banana Juice

Ingredients:

1 cup of cherries, pitted

1 large banana, peeled

1 cup of blueberries

1 whole lemon, peeled

1 small Granny Smith's apple, cored

¼ tsp of cinnamon

Preparation:

Wash the cherries and cut in half. Remove the pits and stems. Set aside.

Peel the banana and cut into small chunks. Set aside.

Rinse the blueberries using a large colander. Drain and set aside.

Peel the lemon and cut lengthwise in half. Set aside.

Wash the apple and cut lengthwise in half. Remove the core and cut into small pieces. Set aside.

Now, combine cherries, banana, blueberries, lemon, and

apple in a juicer and process until juiced. Transfer to a serving glass and stir in the cinnamon.

Add some ice and serve immediately.

Nutrition information per serving: Kcal: 340, Protein: 5.5g, Carbs: 102g, Fats: 1.7g

26. Banana Celery Juice

Ingredients:

1 medium-sized banana, sliced

1 medium-sized celery stalk, chopped

3 whole apricots, chopped

1 small apple, chopped

Preparation:

Peel the banana and cut into small chunks. Set aside.

Wash the celery stalk and cut into bite-sized pieces. Set aside.

Wash the apricots and cut in half. Remove the pits and cut into bite-sized pieces. Set aside.

Wash the apple and cut in half. Remove the core and cut into bite-sized pieces. Set aside.

Now, combine banana, celery, apricots, and apple in a juicer and process until juiced. Transfer to a serving glass and add some ice.

Serve immediately.

Nutrition information per serving: Kcal: 154, Protein: 3.5g, Carbs: 45.8g, Fats: 1.1g

27. Cucumber Onion Juice

Ingredients:

1 cup of cucumber, chopped

1 spring onion, chopped

1 medium-sized tomato, chopped

1 yellow bell pepper, chopped

¼ tsp of Himalayan salt

3 oz of water

Preparation:

Place the tomato in a bowl and cut into quarters. Reserve the tomato juice while cutting and set aside.

Wash the bell pepper and cut in half. Remove the seeds and cut into small pieces. Set aside.

Wash the cucumber and cut into thick slices.

Wash the spring onion and chop it into small pieces. Set aside.

Now, combine cucumber, onion, tomato, and bell pepper in a juicer and process until juiced.

Transfer to a serving glasses and stir in the salt, water, and reserved tomato juice.

Add some ice cubes before serving and enjoy!

Nutrition information per serving: Kcal: 73, Protein: 3.7g, Carbs: 20.1g, Fats: 0.9g

28. Zucchini Leek Juice

Ingredients:

1 medium-sized zucchini, peeled

1 whole leek, chopped

1 large green apple, peeled and seeds removed

1 cups of mustard greens, chopped

1 cup of Brussels sprouts

1 cup of parsnip, sliced

¼ tsp of ginger, ground

Preparation:

Wash the zucchini and cut in half. Scoop out the seeds using a spoon. Cut into small chunks and set aside.

Wash the leek and cut into small pieces. Set aside.

Wash the apple and remove the core. Cut into bite-sized pieces and set aside.

Wash the mustard greens and torn with hands. Set aside.

Wash the Brussels sprouts and trim off the outer leaves. Set aside.

Wash the parsnips and cut into thick slices. Set aside.

Now, process zucchini, leek, apple, mustard greens, Brussels sprouts, and parsnips in a juicer.

Transfer to serving glasses and refrigerate for 10 minutes before serving.

Nutrition information per serving: Kcal: 284, Protein: 12.3g, Carbs: 83.7g, Fats: 2.4g

29. Celery Beet Juice

Ingredients:

1 cup of celery, chopped

1 cup of beets, sliced

1 cup of pomegranate seeds

1 cup of crookneck squash, sliced

1 tbsp of honey

¼ tsp of ginger, ground

Preparation:

Wash the celery and cut into small pieces. Set aside.

Wash the beets and trim off the green parts. Cut into bite-sized pieces and set aside.

Cut the top of the pomegranate fruit using a sharp knife. Slice down to each of the white membranes inside of the fruit. Pop the seeds into a measuring cup and set aside.

Wash the crookneck squash and cut in half. Scoop out the seeds using a spoon. Cut into small chunks and set aside. Reserve the rest for another juice.

Now, process celery, beets, beet greens, pomegranate

seeds, and squash in a juicer.

Transfer to serving glasses and stir in the honey.

Add some ice and serve immediately.

Nutrition information per serving: Kcal: 132, Protein: 6.4g, Carbs: 48.8g, Fats: 1.8g

30. Orange Carrot Juice

Ingredients:

1 large orange, peeled and wedged

1 large carrot, sliced

1 cup of pumpkin, cubed

1 cup of cucumber, sliced

1 small ginger knob, chopped

Preparation:

Peel the orange and divide into wedges. Cut each wedge in half and set aside.

Wash and peel the carrot. Cut into thin slices and set aside.

Cut the top of a pumpkin. Cut lengthwise in half and then scrape out the seeds. Cut one large wedge and peel it. Cut into small cubes and fill the measuring cup. Reserve the rest in the refrigerator.

Wash the cucumber and cut into thin slices. Fill the measuring cup and reserve the rest for later. Set aside.

Peel the ginger knob and cut into small pieces. Set aside.

Now, combine, orange, carrot, pumpkin, cucumber, and ginger in a juicer. Process until well juiced. Transfer to a serving glass and add some ice.

Serve immediately.

Nutrition information per serving: Kcal: 130, Protein: 4.1g, Carbs: 39.1g, Fats: 0.6g

31. Blueberry Lettuce Juice

Ingredients:

1 cup of blueberries

1 cup of Romaine lettuce, shredded

1 whole lime, peeled

1 large banana, sliced

1 whole cucumber, sliced

1 oz of water

Preparation:

Rinse the blueberries using a small colander. Slightly drain and fill the measuring cup. Set aside.

Rinse the lettuce thoroughly under cold running water. Shred it and fill the measuring cup. Set aside.

Peel the lime and cut lengthwise in half. Set aside.

Peel the banana and cut into thin slices. Set aside.

Wash the cucumber and cut into thin slices. Set aside.

Now, combine blueberries, lettuce, lime, banana, and cucumber in a juicer and process until juiced. Transfer to a serving glass and stir in the water. Add some crushed ice and serve immediately.

Nutrition information per serving: Kcal: 176, Protein: 9.8g, Carbs: 49.5g, Fats: 1.7g

32. Basil Avocado Juice

Ingredients:

1 cup of fresh basil, torn

1 cup of avocado, cut into bite-sized pieces

1 cup of cucumber, sliced

1 medium-sized zucchini, chopped

1 cup of red leaf lettuce, torn

Preparation:

Combine basil and lettuce in a large colander and rinse under cold running water. Drain and torn with hands into small pieces. Set aside.

Peel the avocado and cut lengthwise in half. Remove the pit and cut into bite-sized pieces. Fill the measuring cup and reserve the rest in the refrigerator.

Wash the cucumber and cut into thin slices. Fill the measuring cup and refrigerate for later.

Peel the zucchini and chop into small pieces. Set aside.

Now, combine basil, avocado, cucumber, lettuce, and zucchini in a juicer. Process until well juiced. Transfer to a serving glass and add some ice.

Serve immediately.

Nutrition information per serving: Kcal: 234, Protein: 6.7g, Carbs: 21.7g, Fats: 22.3g

33.   Honey Lemon Juice

Ingredients:

1 tbsp honey, raw

1 whole lemon, peeled

1 cup of strawberries, chopped

1 cup of spinach, torn

1 whole lime, peeled

2 oz of water

Preparation:

Peel the lemon and lime. Cut each fruit lengthwise in half and set aside.

Wash the strawberries and remove the stems. Cut into bite-sized pieces and set aside.

Wash the spinach thoroughly under cold running water. Slightly drain and torn into small pieces. Set aside.

Now, combine spinach, lemon, lime, and strawberries in a juicer and process until juiced. Transfer to a serving glass and stir in the water and honey.

Refrigerate for 5 minutes before serving.

Enjoy!

Nutrition information per serving: Kcal: 81, Protein: 5.8g, Carbs: 27.8g, Fats: 1.4g

34. Cantaloupe Cucumber Juice

Ingredients:

1 cup of cantaloupe, diced

1 medium-sized cucumber, peeled

1 cup of baby spinach, torn

1 cup of cranberries

1 cup of parsley, chopped

1 tbsp of honey, raw

Preparation:

Cut the cantaloupe in half. Scoop out the seeds and flesh. Cut two wedges and peel them. Chop into chunks and set aside. Reserve the rest of the cantaloupe in a refrigerator.

Wash the cucumber and cut into thick slices. Set aside.

Combine spinach and parsley in a colander and wash under cold running water. Torn with hands and set aside.

Wash the cranberries and set aside.

Now, process cantaloupe, cucumber, parsley, baby spinach, and cranberries in a juicer.

Transfer to serving glasses and stir in the honey.

Refrigerate for 5 minutes before serving.

Enjoy!

Nutrition information per serving: Kcal: 197, Protein: 10.2g, Carbs: 58.3g, Fats: 2.2g

35. Cinnamon Peach Juice

Ingredients:

¼ tsp of cinnamon, ground

1 large peach, pitted and chopped

1 small green apple, cored and chopped

1 whole banana, sliced

1 oz of coconut water

1 tbsp of mint, finely chopped

Preparation:

Wash the peach and cut lengthwise in half. Remove the pit and cut into bite-sized pieces. Set side.

Wash the apple and cut in half. Remove the core and chop into small pieces. Set aside.

Peel the banana and cut into thin slices. Set aside.

Now, combine peach, apple, and bananas in a juicer and process until well juiced. Transfer to a serving glass and stir in the cinnamon and coconut water.

Sprinkle with mint and add ice.

Enjoy!

Nutrition information per serving: Kcal: 362, Protein: 5.5g, Carbs: 104g, Fats: 1.7g

36. Avocado Ginger Juice

Ingredients:

1 cup of avocado, chopped

1 small ginger knob

1 cup of beets, trimmed

1 large carrot, sliced

¼ tsp turmeric, ground

2 oz water

Preparation:

Peel the avocado and cut lengthwise in half. Remove the pit and cut into bite-sized pieces. Fill the measuring cup and reserve the rest in the refrigerator.

Peel the ginger knob and cut into small pieces. Set aside.

Trim off the green parts of the beets. Slightly peel and cut into thin slices. Fill the measuring cup and refrigerate the rest.

Wash and peel the carrot. Cut into bite-sized pieces and set aside.

Now, combine avocado, ginger, beets, and carrot in a

juicer. Process until well juiced and transfer to a serving glass. Stir in the turmeric and water and refrigerate for 5 minutes before serving.

Enjoy!

Nutrition information per serving: Kcal: 265, Protein: 5.9g, Carbs: 33.4g, Fats: 21.8g

37. Asparagus Cucumber Juice

Ingredients:

1 cup of asparagus, chopped

1 cup of cucumber, sliced

1 cup of cauliflower, chopped

1 cup of celery, chopped

¼ tsp of turmeric, ground

Preparation:

Wash the asparagus under cold running water. Trim off the woody ends and chop into bite-sized pieces. Set aside.

Wash the cucumber and cut into thin slices. Fill the measuring cup and reserve the rest in the refrigerator.

Wash the cauliflower and trim off the outer leaves. Chop into small pieces and fill the measuring cup. Reserve the rest for later.

Wash the celery and chop into bite-sized pieces. Set aside.

Now, combine asparagus, cucumber, cauliflower, and celery in a juicer and process until juiced. Transfer to a serving glass and stir in the turmeric.

Serve immediately.

Nutrition information per serving: Kcal: 52, Protein: 6.1g, Carbs: 15.4g, Fats: 0.7g

38. Salted Avocado Juice

Ingredients:

1 cup of avocado, cubed

1 cup of celery, chopped

3 large radishes, chopped

1 small zucchini, sliced

1 cup of cucumber, sliced

¼ tsp of salt

1 oz of water

Preparation:

Peel the avocado and cut in half. Remove the pit and cut into small cubes. Fill the measuring cup and reserve the rest for later.

Wash the celery and chop it into bite-sized pieces. Set aside.

Wash the radishes and cut into small pieces. Set aside.

Wash the zucchini and cut into thin slices. Set aside.

Wash the cucumber and cut into thin slices. Fill the

measuring cup and reserve the rest for later. Set aside.

Now, combine avocado, celery, radishes, zucchini, and cucumber in a juicer and process until juiced. Transfer to a serving glass and stir in the salt and water.

Serve cold.

Nutrition information per serving: Kcal: 235, Protein: 5.6g, Carbs: 22.3g, Fats: 22.6g

39.   Kiwi Apple Juice

Ingredients:

2 whole kiwis, peeled and halved

1 medium-sized Granny Smith's apple, cored

3 whole apricots, chopped

1 large banana, chunked

Preparation:

Peel the kiwi and cut lengthwise in half. Set aside.

Wash the apple and cut lengthwise in half. Remove the core and cut into bite-sized pieces. Set aside.

Wash the apricots and cut in half. Remove the pits and cut into small pieces. Set aside.

Peel the banana and cut into small chunks. Set aside.

Now, combine kiwi, apple, apricots, and banana in a juicer and process until juiced. Transfer to a serving glass and add some ice.

Serve immediately.

Nutrition information per serving: Kcal: 313, Protein: 5.4g, Carbs: 91g, Fats: 1.9g

40. Kale Parsley Juice

Ingredients:

1 cup of kale, chopped

2 cups of parsley, chopped

1 whole grapefruit, peeled

1 cup of watermelon, diced

2 oz of water

Preparation:

Wash the kale and parsley under cold running water. Torn with hands and set aside.

Peel the grapefruit and cut into small pieces. Set aside.

Cut the watermelon lengthwise. For one cup, you will need about 1 large wedge. Peel and cut into chunks. Remove the seeds and set aside. Reserve the rest of the melon for some other juices.

Now, process kale, parsley, grapefruit, watermelon in a juicer. Transfer to serving glasses and stir in the water.

Add some ice and serve immediately.

Nutrition information per serving: Kcal: 161, Protein: 6.4g, Carbs: 45.6g, Fats: 1.5g

41. Ginger Pepper Juice

Ingredients:

¼ tsp of ginger, ground

1 large red bell pepper, chopped

1 cup of cauliflower, chopped

1 cup of Brussels sprouts, halved

2 oz of water

Preparation:

Trim off the outer leaves of a cauliflower. Wash it and cut into small pieces. Fill the measuring cup and reserve the rest in the refrigerator.

Wash the Brussels sprouts and trim off the wilted layers. Cut each in half and fill the measuring cup. Set aside.

Wash the bell pepper and cut lengthwise in half. Remove the seeds and the top stem. Cut into small pieces and set aside.

Now, combine pepper, cauliflower, and Brussels sprouts in a juicer and process until juiced. Transfer to a serving glass and stir in the water and ginger.

Serve immediately.

Nutrition information per serving: Kcal: 106, Protein: 9.6g, Carbs: 30.9g, Fats: 1.3g

42. Coconut Kale Juice

Ingredients:

1 cup of fresh kale, chopped

1 oz of coconut water

1 large banana, peeled and chunked

1 small Granny Smith's apple, cored

1 cup of Brussels sprouts, halved

¼ tsp of ginger, ground

Preparation:

Wash the kale thoroughly under cold running water and slightly drain. Chop into small pieces and set aside.

Peel the banana and cut into small chunks. Set aside.

Wash the apple and cut in half. Remove the core and cut into bite-sized pieces. Set aside.

Wash the Brussels sprouts and remove the outer wilted layers. Cut each in half and set aside.

Now, combine kale, banana, apple, and Brussels sprouts in a juicer and process until juiced. Transfer to a serving glass and stir in the coconut water and ginger.

Add some ice and serve immediately.

Nutrition information per serving: Kcal: 223, Protein: 7.9g, Carbs: 64.4g, Fats: 1.6g

43. Lemon Beet Juice

Ingredients:

1 whole lemon, peeled

1 cup of beets, sliced

1 cup of raspberries

1 medium-sized pear, chopped

1 oz of water

Preparation:

Peel the lemon and cut lengthwise in half. Set aside.

Wash the beets and trim off the green parts. Cut into thin slices and fill the measuring cup. Reserve the rest for later.

Rinse well the raspberries using a small colander. Drain and set aside.

Wash the pear and cut in half. Remove the core and cut into bite-sized pieces. Set aside.

Now, combine lemon, beets, raspberries, and pear in a juicer and process until juiced. Transfer to a serving glass and stir in the water.

Refrigerate for 5 minutes before serving.

Nutrition information per serving: Kcal: 165, Protein: 4.9g, Carbs: 60.2g, Fats: 1.4g

44. Blackberry Pineapple Juice

Ingredients:

1 cup of blackberries

1 cup of pineapple, chunked

1 whole lime, peeled

1 large banana, sliced

2 oz of water

Preparation:

Place the blackberries in a small colander and wash under cold running water. Slightly drain and set aside.

Using a sharp paring knife, cut the top of the pineapple. Gently remove all hard skin and slice it into thin slices. Fill the measuring cup and reserve the rest for later.

Peel the banana and cut into thin slices. Set aside.

Peel the lime and cut lengthwise in half. Set aside.

Now, combine blackberries, pineapple, banana, and lime in a juicer. Process until well juiced. Transfer to a serving glass and add some ice before serving.

Enjoy!

Nutrition information per serving: Kcal: 222, Protein: 4.5g, Carbs: 70.2g, Fats: 1.4g

45. Watercress Rosemary Juice

Ingredients:

1 cup of watercress, torn

1 rosemary sprig, finely chopped

1 medium whole tomato, chopped

1 large red bell pepper, chopped

1 oz of water

Preparation:

Wash the watercress thoroughly under cold running water. Slightly drain and torn with hands into small pieces. Set aside.

Wash the tomato and place in a small bowl. Chop into small pieces and make sure to reserve the tomato juice while cutting. Set aside.

Wash the bell pepper and cut lengthwise in half. Remove the seeds and chop into small pieces. Set aside.

Now, combine watercress, bell pepper, and tomato in a juicer and process until juiced. Transfer to a serving glass and stir in the water and reserved tomato juice.

Sprinkle with rosemary and serve immediately.

Enjoy!

Nutrition information per serving: Kcal: 56, Protein: 3.5g, Carbs: 15.1g, Fats: 0.7g

46.   Carrot Apple Juice

Ingredients:

1 large carrot, sliced

1 small Red Delicious apple, cored

1 cup of celery, chopped

1 whole lemon, peeled

¼ tsp ginger, ground

1 oz of water

Preparation:

Wash and peel the carrot. Cut into small slices and set aside.

Wash the apple and cut in half. Remove the core and cut into bite-sized pieces. Set aside.

Wash the celery and cut into small pieces. Set aside.

Peel the lemon and cut lengthwise in half. Set aside.

Now, combine carrot, apple, celery, and lemon in a juicer and process until juiced. Transfer to a serving glass and stir in the water and ginger. If you like, add some crushed ice.

Serve immediately.

Nutrition information per serving: Kcal: 105, Protein: 2.4g, Carbs: 32.8g, Fats: 0.7g

47. Spinach Swiss Chard Juice

Ingredients:

1 cup of fresh spinach, chopped

1 cup of Swiss chard, torn

1 cup of cucumber, sliced

1 cup of fresh kale, chopped

¼ tsp of ginger, ground

1 oz of water

Preparation:

Combine spinach, kale, and Swiss chard in a large colander. Rinse under cold running water and slightly drain. Chop all into small pieces and set aside.

Wash the cucumber and cut into thin slices. Fill the measuring cup and reserve the rest in the refrigerator.

Now, combine spinach, Swiss chard, cucumber, and kale in a juicer and process until well juiced. Transfer to a serving glass and stir in the ginger and water.

Refrigerate before serving.

Enjoy!

Nutrition information per serving: Kcal: 63, Protein: 9.9g, Carbs: 16.7g, Fats: 1.6g

48. Spinach Tomato Juice

Ingredients:

1 cup of fresh spinach, torn

1 medium-sized tomato, chopped

1 cup of purple cabbage, chopped

1 cup of beets, sliced

1 large red bell pepper, chopped

¼ tsp of salt

Preparation:

Combine spinach and cabbage in a large colander. Rinse thoroughly under cold running water and drain. Torn into small pieces and set aside.

Wash the tomato and chop into small pieces. Set aside.

Wash the beets and trim off the green parts. Peel and cut into thin slices and fill the measuring cup. Reserve the rest for later.

Wash the bell pepper and cut lengthwise in half. Remove the stem and seeds. Cut into small pieces and set aside.

Now, combine spinach, tomatoes, cabbage, beets, and

bell pepper in a juicer and process until juiced. Transfer to a serving glass and stir in the salt.

Serve immediately.

Nutrition information per serving: Kcal: 134, Protein: 11.5g, Carbs: 39.1g, Fats: 1.8g

49. Carrot Fennel Juice

Ingredients:

1 medium-sized carrot, sliced

1 medium-sized fennel bulb

1 small ginger knob, peeled

½ cup of cabbage, torn

2 oz of water

Preparation:

Wash and peel the carrot. Cut into thin slices and set aside.

Wash the fennel and trim off the green ends. Using a sharp paring knife, remove the outer layer. Cut into small pieces and set aside.

Peel the ginger knob and cut into small pieces. Set aside.

Wash the cabbage thoroughly and torn into small pieces. Set aside.

Now, combine carrot, fennel, ginger, and cabbage in a juicer and process until juiced. Transfer to a serving glass and stir in the water. Refrigerate before serving.

Enjoy!

Nutrition information per serving: Kcal: 72, Protein: 4g, Carbs: 25.9g, Fats: 0.7g

ADDITIONAL TITLES FROM THIS AUTHOR

70 Effective Meal Recipes to Prevent and Solve Being Overweight: Burn Fat Fast by Using Proper Dieting and Smart Nutrition

By Joe Correa CSN

48 Acne Solving Meal Recipes: The Fast and Natural Path to Fixing Your Acne Problems in Less Than 10 Days!

By Joe Correa CSN

41 Alzheimer's Preventing Meal Recipes: Reduce or Eliminate Your Alzheimer's Condition in 30 Days or Less!

By Joe Correa CSN

70 Effective Breast Cancer Meal Recipes: Prevent and Fight Breast Cancer with Smart Nutrition and Powerful Foods

By Joe Correa CSN

www.ingramcontent.com/pod-product-compliance
Lightning Source LLC
Chambersburg PA
CBHW030257030426
42336CB00009B/421